How I Navigate My Health Maintenance Organization

James Nugent

Disclaimer

I am not a doctor or a lawyer. This booklet is not meant as medical or legal advice. It is just a recounting of my personal experiences and my personal philosophy which guide me. Your opinions may differ.

Introduction

I was born in the early 1960's. The was a radically new approach to health available in the Puget Sound region at that time. I was one of the first 51,000 people to become a member of Group Health Cooperative of Puget Sound. Although it was actually my parents that registered me at my birth as a member; it would shape my view of health care and to a certain extent life.

What is a doctor for?

In 1992 I was directing a summer program held at the University of Washington campus. It was an English/Chinese Language institute. I spoke with a participant who had a very strong view concerning health care. She said that in China people pay a monthly fee to a general practitioner doctor whom only gets paid if you are well.

If you fall ill the doctor has failed. In China a good doctor protects your health and keeps you from getting sick.

I found the above concept improbable and yet something seemed familiar to me. The Chinese were the same people who (in Taiwan) do not let you move into a privately owned apartment (a condominium) until you have completely paid for it! They are very practical in the way they consume health care and the way they extend credit.

Perhaps there is something backward or impractical in how we consume medical services. Most people only go to the doctor after they are sick. Maybe it is wiser to prevent problems with your health rather than react to a health crisis.

Toward a More Proactive Lifestyle

I have generally tried to stay out of hospitals and away from doctors. I associate them with pain, sickness and death. However, I have been forced by circumstances over the last quarter to reevaluate this common attitude. The change in attitude probably has prolonged my life.

The following stories are specifically about my HMO which is called Group Health Cooperative of Puget Sound or GHC. The services provided by every HMO will be different. However, until you start exploring what your HMO provides and how you access; it can't do a lot of good for you.

The Fourth of July

I stepped on a rusty nail while taking apart my sundeck. I had advised many other people to check with their doctor when they got injured, but it was hard for me to call GHC 24-hour consulting nurse.

All I wanted to know was if I needed to go get a tetanus shot. Late in the day, I called the nurse and didn't know what to say. I started with, "I did something stupid…" She interrupted me and said in a cheerful voice, "Of course, you did. It is The fourth of July!" I laughed and was put at ease. She had instant access to my records and determined that I needed to get a shot. I just needed to go across town in the morning and walk into the urgent care facility.

I went to the urgent care facility. There were no patients waiting so I was ushered right in. In the injection room a young female nurse and an even younger newbie got my shot ready.

At the last second I asked to lie down, and have somebody with gray hair do the actual shot. Everybody laughed including me and I was escorted to a bunk. An elderly gray haired male nurse came in smiling and gave me a painless injection. I was out of there in less than 5 minutes.

Using a Consulting Nurse.

I no longer procrastinate when I need to decide about going to the doctor. I just call the consulting nurse and get the facts about my condition. Sometimes I have been told to go to urgent care or my doctor immediately and other times I have been told to watch and see. If I need to go see my doctor now, she can make an appointment with the doctor for me.

More Information Is available

I can ask a medical question of a consulting nurse or I can read about thousands of medical issues by going to the GHC website. I use the website about three times a year. I have visited the website often in recent years, partially because I have had a lot of tests and meetings with various assorted specialists. Also it is just interesting to learn about medical stuff.

When I make an appointment with a doctor, I try to be a little knowledgeable so we can talk about my medical issues. Otherwise I am just going to be completely dependent on what he/she knows and thinks. Like going to a mechanic; I would just have to accept whatever the doctor said.

I feel that as an HMO consumer I need to take an active part in decisions about my health care. This also forces my doctor to consult with other doctors when he or she doesn't know something! In most situations I actually have an entire team of experts working with me when needed.

Communication is the Key

I am free to contact my anybody on my health care team 24-hours a day via e-mail. I get a response by the next day. Sometimes if the doctor has something complex to say or ask, he will actually call me on the phone.

Referrals

My doctor usually makes the referrals for other services if I agree. However, I can self-refer to almost any medical provider inside the cooperative and sometimes outside if necessary.

Appointments are usually just a week or two away. Copays on services are generally $20 a visit.

Medications

Most of my medicines have copays of $5 for a 90-day supply. I can order my meds by phone, internet or in person.

I am in the driver's seat.

I am complete control in how I am treated and who treats me. On rare occasions I have not liked the way somebody has treated me. I have a right to lodge a complaint. I can also just change doctors. I have done both.

GHC is not like going to my mechanic. When I take my car to the mechanic; I just tell him what I think is wrong and he fixes it. Hopefully it is cheap and I don't have to visit for long time.

My HMO is a partnership. I don't have to do what the experts say but it is usually foolish not to take their advice seriously. For example, statin drugs until recently were generally prescribed for people with my medical history.

I was happy to comply because it seemed to make sense. When I started taking the drug it had harsh side effects. I restarted the drug twice more. Each time it was quickly intolerable. Since my cholesterol and blood fats were semi normal I told my doctor that I would not taking the drug at this time. He noted it in my file and that was the end of that. We will revisit the issue if my hyperlipidemia returns.

Health Promotion and Disease Prevention (HPDP)

HPDP is really a big part of the services at Group Health Cooperative. Every year GHC e-mails when it is time for my flu shot and diagnostic blood samples and other procedures. They also review my computerized file and notify me when my inoculations are due. They have a free gym membership benefit for elderly cooperative members. The have free and cheap classes and support groups for diet and diabetes and numerous other health issues. The healthier you are the less you will cost the organization. It turns out that it costs a lot less to prevent a health problem than treat a health problem!

Some people find this kind of health care too intrusive but actually sometimes we all need a little help starting a sensitive discussion with somebody who has the resources to help. So I get asked now and then to come to my doctor's office just for a free blood pressure check. Sometimes when I am visiting for check-up, I am asked to fill out a general survey. I seem to remember them asking me about drinking, smoking, suicidal ideation, and maybe seatbelts. It is all self-reported stuff but research shows that people will often disclose when they have a problem. It is interesting to note that they charge a higher monthly fee for the insurance for everyone in the family if you smoke. The whole point is to reduce your suffering and their cost.

How my HMO works, for me.

Beside all the preventative lifestyle opportunities; they have responded immediately to my various health problems. Thirty years ago a GHC physician's assistant did his best to encourage me to lose a little weight. Ten years after that I was 20 pounds even heavier.

I was sitting on a sofa on a Saturday afternoon and I noticed a one-inch tall bump on my forearm. We are Catholics, so I asked my wife to pray over the lump and it shrank in just a few moments. Still it was still slightly visible. We believe God can work through doctors too, so I called the consulting nurse and she made an appointment for me. Monday morning, I was seeing my doctor who looked at the tiny lump and quickly said it was nothing to worry about. While I was there she asked me to make an appointment for a check-up and get a basic blood panel. I walked down stairs and had my blood drawn. Wednesday the doctor's office called me and said that I had diabetes and other problems with my blood samples. The nurse asked if I could I come in immediately and start treatment? Within 6 weeks: diet, prayer, exercise, and GHC made me well again. I needed no meds and had no problems with my blood chemistry. If I had not actively participated in the process and done it my way, I doubt I wouldn't even be alive. My father died when he was 49 and I do not think that he effectively took responsibility for his health.

They whole story of my recovery is told in detail in another small book called "Miracle in Young Cove." It is available at Amazon.com

GHC Working for Me Again

Three years ago, I was thirty pounds, over-weight. My blood pressure soared to 210/110. Normal blood pressure in considered 120/80. My blood pressure was extremely dangerous. I had a stroke and lost my ability to speak clearly.

I met my new doctor in the local urgent care facility. He released me to my nearby home after I was somewhat stabilized. He prescribed several different medications and I talked to him by phone or email every 12 hours. I monitored my blood pressure and as the weeks went by it came down to 170/95 Then we began searching for the cause of the high blood pressure. We explored all sort of rare causes. I saw several specialists.

Last month we discovered that sleep apnea was the cause of my high blood pressure. After only 2 weeks on a breathing machine at night; my blood pressure dropped to 148/84. It turns out that I would stop breathing 16 times an hour. With the machine helping me breath, I am now normal.

My doctor's office monitors my breathing occasionally via a cell phone connection with the shoebox size machine at my bedside. I will live! A detailed account of this three-year medical mystery will be available at Amazon.com this summer. It is called, "Without Air" by James Nugent.

What keeps people from taking control of their health?

Well, if we are looking for an excuse, we could blame our entire culture. As a nation we usually only see a doctor when we can't deny that something is wrong. Even stroke victims and heart attack victims will delay getting help until it is too late.

My Stroke

I awakened on a Monday morning after a mild stroke and just figured that I couldn't talk because I had nasal congestion and postnasal drip. This was my excuse for not going for help; at least until noon!

Fear

Fear is another reason people don't take charge. It is irrational but people avoid the doctor because of what doctors do to their bodies.

Some procedures are embarrassing and some our painful. A gynecological exam or a prostate exam are yucky but absolutely necessary and potentially life-saving.

Somethings hurt a little or a lot. I have phobia of needles that compelled me to leave a dentist's office and did not return to a dentist for 13 years. I didn't return to a new dentist until I had broken a tooth. Then it was discovered that I had gum disease and several problems that required three caps and several fillings. It also cost about $3000.

If only I had taken a proactive strategy with my dental health, as I have taken with the rest of my health! I now go my dentists every 6 months and doing all I should to prevent problems. Getting over my fear with the dentist has also helped me deal with needles at GHC.

Hypochondria

Before you start reading about all the diseases and ailments on your HMO website, get a thorough check-up with a doctor you trust. Then when you read about all the ills; you will be less convinced that you are going to die from something.

This phenomena, is very real and disturbing for some people. When I was in graduate school for my Master's degree in counseling, I met several normal students who became convinced that there we secretly stark raving mad. They had to go to counseling just to convince them that they were ok! If you learn about medical problems; there is a chance that you may think for a time that you have something wrong.

Keeping Your Own Records

If you are going to be in charge of your health you will want to keep logs of your health. For example, I monitor my blood pressure twice a day. Since high blood pressure has been a serious issue, I wanted to see if it fluctuates daily or weekly. I noticed that it did change in response to various meds. Eventually this helped my doctor and I figure out a way to keep me alive until we found the cause of my problem.

I am told that they never find the cause of high blood pressure in 80% of the patients, but we had to find out because it was extreme. My doctor and I have the same philosophy. We use the least amount of medicine to get the job done.

I also keep track of a variety blood chemistry issues every three months. I monitor things like: A1c (blood sugar), cholesterol, triglycerides and such. I have several home testing devices.

These serve as an early warning protocol and gives me peace of mind. I would e-mail my doctor if there was anything alarming. All is well so far.

While all the lab testing at GHC is quite accurate and adequate for my safety; I also use my home data to help me refine my diet and exercise program. For example, I found that everything stays stable and healthy if I exercise an hour a day. Half an hour doesn't do it and 90 minutes doesn't seem to help to any greater degree.

I read somewhere that one should not check there weight every day. I do, and keep track. It helps me stay focused on weight loss. I celebrate even little wins. Yes, it fluctuates in little bit everyday but I can see the general trend over time.

Once in a great while all this DIY data collection actually gives my health care team a clue about what we might do to help me.

The number one issue I am facing right now is that I am fat. If I lost 30 pounds; it might mean that I live a long and interesting life. I have found a diet plan that works for me. It turns out that the American Diabetes Association has a diet that is well tested an easy for me to do.

I can stay on it for the rest of my life and it is not very restrictive. I like it. I met with a GHC dietitian and that was helpful too.

For years I have failed to lose weight. I am very optimistic now.

Healthy Tips

I have spent enough time in healthcare facilities to develop a few tips for preserving your health. Yep, there are a very high concentration of sick people in healthcare facilities. I would hate to catch some horrible disease when I go to the hospitable.

1. Think positively. Worry can lower your immunity.

2. Wash your hands before and after your visit.

3. Try not to touch surfaces that other patients touch.

4. Don't touch your: eyes, nose or mouth.

5. Make sure your doctor washes their hands.

6. Stay out of the elevator.

7. Stay out of the restroom if possible.

8. Sit well away from anybody with a cough.

9. Bring your own pen.

10. Remember, you are in charge of your health.

So where do I start?

I would read the actual agreement which controls what happens at your HMO. Find out what services it will provide and what services it will not. You may find to your dismay that something you want is not adequately provided.

For example, what is the outpatient benefit for mental health? You may find that it your present HMO provides no services for Adult Children of Alcoholics. Or maybe there are no maternity services. If your HMO does not meet your needs what good is it? Find a HMO that meets your needs.

Then find out how you access the HMO services.

Attitude

Go with a positive attitude and be kind to the healthcare providers. They are people too! I find that what goes around comes around.

Remember to get full service from you HMO you must be a full participant.

Don't view your healthcare as something you must fight for. You are already in charge and you have real experts on your side.

Take full advantage of all the health promotion and disease prevention of your HMO.

Words of Wisdom in a Poem

We are what we are

We do what we do

We are nothing less

And nothing more

Than what we choose to be…

JJ N

It is my sincere hope that your HMO will keep you healthy and happy through your life. I have found that when people are angry or disappointed with my MHO; they simple didn't understand their role on their healthcare team.

A Joke and a Lesson

Q. What's the difference between a doctor and God?

A. God knows He is not a doctor :>

Lesson

Not at my HMO. My doctor is my quarterback on my team.

Best Regards

James Nugent

4-15-16

Books by James Nugent

How I Navigate My Health Maintenance Organization

Catholic Way of Suffering

A Moment Before Sunrise

Teaching Anger Management to Elementary Students

E-book Writing and My Search for Inspiration

The Joy of Cats

Thank You

Living on the Edge of Civilization

Adventures on the Olympia Harbor Patrol

How I Sailed from Olympia to the San Juan Islands, and Returned Safely

An Alternative Boating Guide to Southern Puget Sound

Twenty Hours under the Sea

Without Speech

Miracles in Young Cove

Home Self-defense

How and Why I lived Aboard

Kayaking Budd Inlet in South Puget Sound

Writing E-books and Making the Perfect Book

I Speak Esperanto

The Rainbow Road and Other Signs of God's Love

Write a Book

Living an Abundant Life, Within Your Means

Crazy Making

Social Jujitsu and Powerful Principles for Managing Social Conflict

Advanced Social Jujitsu

Blackjack on My Small Budget

A Little Benedictine Oblate Manuel

Without Speech

All things work

Loving Time with Your Creator

Personal Adventures in a Life of Learning

Loving Time with Your Creator

The Good News about Being Catholic

The Extraordinary Eucharistic Visitor

E-book Writing and Overcoming Barriers to Creativity

Living an Abundant Life Within Your Means

E-book Writing and Organizing Your Ideas

Paddling to the Rhythm of God

My Forty Days for Life 2013

Lifestyle Reality Observing

How to Sail in the Winter

How to Get Your Kid to Move Out

How to Get What Want

Sex, Abstinence, and Happiness

Cynthia Says Radio Show – Anger is a choice

Eight Things You Need to Survive

Three Moms from Hell

Moving and Starting Fresh

More Good News about Being Catholic

The Solo Kayak

Everyday Survival Kit

Rainy Day Kayak

Night Kayak

Solo Kayak II

Paddles and Water

A Beach Naturalist on Southern Puget Sound

Clean House Clean Life

The Total Catholic Christian

Advanced Social Jujitsu

The Beginning School Counselor

Managing the Most Difficult Students

Not Taking Responsibility

The Friends You Keep

Happiness is a Choice

Why Write?

The Voyages of Saint Bernadett

Available at Amazon.com in Kindle E-Book and or Audible Book or Paperback

Notes

www.ingramcontent.com/pod-product-compliance
Lightning Source LLC
Chambersburg PA
CBHW070838310526
45788CB00017B/2065